ZEN
AND THE
ART of SLEEP

Eric Chiles

© 2009 by Eric Chiles

For more information contact Pilatus Publishing
P.O. Box 82724 Austin, TX 78708

ISBN 978-0-9723950-3-8
LCCN 2008935449

This book is dedicated to my sister,
who shares my longing
for life's more substantial truths.

Contents

To carry yourself forward and experience myraid things

is delusion;

That myraid things come forth and experience themselves

is awakening.

Dogen, Genjo Koan

Preface

At first, his words were hard to make out in the bustle of customers and the clatter of dishes in that downtown coffee shop. My Zen Buddhist friend and I were discussing insomnia: I was describing my nightly struggle to get to sleep, and how insomnia had been making my life miserable for several years.

He listened patiently at first, expressing his usual sympathy, then gradually became annoyed. Finally, he stared at me and said, "Why don't you just stop trying so hard, and let sleep do whatever it does?"

My initial reaction was to smile, roll my eyes upwards in a "here-we-go-again" expression, and automatically dismiss his suggestion. I often did that when he dropped bits of his Zen philosophy into our conversations. I never really gave them serious consideration, because frankly my friend's happy-go-lucky attitude had always seemed naive to me. But this time, for some reason, he struck a chord.

Maybe it was because I was becoming utterly desperate to find some relief from the misery of insomnia that impacted so much of my life. I had tried prescription sleeping pills, followed all the advice my doctors gave me, and read every book on sleep I could get my hands on. Nothing had worked.

Was it sheer exhaustion that made me do a mental double-take that day, to sit up and take notice of something I otherwise would have ignored? "Stop trying what?" I asked my friend, my cynicism in temporary remission.

"To control sleep," he replied.

At first, I denied that I was trying to control anything: I suffered from insomnia, which is a medical condition requiring treatment. He just smiled and changed the subject, frustrating me again with this unwillingness to elaborate. So I challenged him again to explain how I was trying to control sleep. That was easy: he just simply repeated back to me everything I had tried. By the time we got our check, it was obvious that my friend was correct. Everything I had done thus far was, in hindsight, an attempt to control sleep. I was trying to make it happen in a certain way and at a certain time.

Here in front of me was an idea that had never occurred to me before: why not just stop trying to control sleep, and let it do whatever it does? It sounded too simple to take seriously — and at the same time, it was too profound to ignore. All of my energy had been focused for so long on obtaining sleep that the option to "Stop trying" didn't even register. It simply did not fit my view of the situation.

Was this really the direction I wanted to take? I thought back over the many times my friend had tried to explain Zen Buddhism to me. My understanding was rather limited, but I knew that the approach somehow favored direct experience over intellectual pursuit. Dissatisfaction and suffering are said to originate from the mind's insistence that the reality of the present moment be something other that what it is. Enlightenment, a concept I'd never given any credence, was obtained by directly apprehending this cause of suffering and thereby becoming free from the mind's tyranny. The mind is what torments us in the first place — or so said the Buddha.

As I sat there staring into my empty coffee cup, considering the possibility that such a hands-off approach might merit further investigation, something profound happened. There was a moment when everything fell into place. For a brief instant, on a very deep level, everything my friend said made complete sense. Sleep *is* whatever it *is*, and *does* whatever it *does*. It was *I* who'd been making sleep into a struggle — not sleep. A great sense of relief swept over me. Here was my answer.

By having no expectations of it, I could render sleep problem-free! Here was an insight I wanted to package and carry with me for the rest of my life. Without realizing it, my mind had instantly reverted to its old ways: I was again thinking about sleep as something to control, or at least influence, using The New Hands-Off Plan. The more my brain kicked into high gear to map out my new strategy, the more my flash of understanding faded away. Try as I might to recapture it, I could not.

However, something felt fundamentally different. As we left the coffee shop in silence, my Buddhist friend sensed that I had glimpsed something extremely important and that I was struggling to fathom it. We both knew that this was neither a matter of him giving advice, nor of my following a set of instructions. The point was for me to see it all clearly once again, this time for more than just a split second.

On the following day I called in sick to my workplace. At the library, with a pile of books on Zen Buddhism stacked in front of me, I began my quest to recapture that insight. Most of what I found was too complicated and abstruse to be of real use, and nowhere in Zen literature could I find anything specifically about sleep. I was frustrated and looking for guidance out of sheer habit, while Zen kept telling me there was no such thing. Slowly it began to dawn on me what the authors were trying to convey. It was my responsibility to look closely at the true nature of my problem without any preconceptions: in the moment of seeing it clearly, there would be peace. If I wanted to understand sleep, then I must learn to view it accurately, without the obstructions of my emotions or intellect.

At first it was puzzling to read the Zen writers' discourse on "seeing clearly," a different way of understanding that was not intellectual or academic. All of it sounded so peculiar. If the true nature of sleep (or, for that matter, anything else) could not be captured with concepts or explanations, how else could it be understood? It surprised me to realize, for the first time, that there exists a deeper sense of truth outside reason and the reasoning process itself. Words cannot describe it, yet this kind of understanding is possible.

Over the course of several months, I began to discover for myself the true nature of sleep. As my comfort level grew with allowing slumber to "be what it is and do what it does," the demands of my will and intellect to control it diminished. In fact, the more I rejected my conceptual explanations of sleep in favor of a direct experience of it, the easier sleep became.

Eventually it was possible to fully grasp what insomnia actually is: an unnecessary form of suffering originating from one's own efforts to obtain sleep. All insomniacs know this important fact on a gut level, even if they are unable to articulate it. Most realize that, if it were just possible to stop trying so hard, then sleep would come naturally. Yet relinquishing our efforts seems impossible when we're laboring under the burden of sleepless nights. Our very nature is to struggle for whatever we believe we need, and, inevitably, the answer is Get More Sleep, a single-minded objective that takes on a life of its own. In the process, we lay our own trap.

The way out of this trap begins with an understanding of why we struggle in the first place. How the mind really works, and, moreover, how to accept its ways, are things that must be learned. Zen Buddhism offers us a framework for that undertaking.

And this is only half the picture. The other half is slumber, of course, which reveals herself only to those with clear vision, unobstructed by the mind's frantic attempts to capture her. My own realization of this mysterious correspondence came after suddenly comprehending some of the key aspects of sleep; these will be discussed in subsequent chapters. Why didn't I notice these facets of sleep before? Because I was too busy thinking! The light comes on when the mind quiets down. This is the path to enlightenment.

The possibility of writing a book to chronicle my own path towards sleep-enlightenment never occurred to me in those early days of my journey. My priority was simply to understand my own sleep on a level that made it less troublesome. Because

this path is essentially one where the mind is quiet, there is no opportunity to actually document anything. How does one describe the nature of sleep without employing the intellect's version of it? It's like trying to use words to describe Van Gogh's "Starry Night," when it really must be *seen* to be appreciated.

Later, though, I felt compelled to share what I'd discovered, and therein lay my challenge: how could I describe something that exists outside words and concepts? If sleep were some *thing* that could easily be defined and put into practice, there would be no problem in the first place. Slumber would have been rendered problem-free long ago. But the real nature of sleep makes this a completely different game. Therefore, if it was not going to be possible for me to recount the true nature of sleep, then perhaps I could at least record the discoveries I made along the way. But could they be understood by others? And finally, my path will not be the same as another individual's path: I had to realize and accept that what works for me might not necessarily work for others.

To uncritically assume that I could somehow light the way for others on the path to satisfying sleep felt not only egotistical, but also risky. A Zen approach is about experiencing reality free from any distortions; that is what gradually taught me to experience sleep on its own terms. My attempt to show others the true nature of sleep could only influence and thereby distort their own understanding. They might be distracted from their own experience by what I wrote, or immediately try to formulate a strategy from it, as I had initially done — in other words, never really look for themselves.

I have concluded that, in order to assist others in understanding their sleep problems as I have understood my own, my task must be limited to helping quiet the intellect and removing any barriers that obstruct the precise observation of one's situation. Such an endeavor cannot be a book about me. It must be a book about you. Or more precisely, what you the reader believe about sleep, perhaps in ways that obscure its true nature. That is what this rather modest little book is all about.

To the extent that self-knowledge is at the heart of Zen, some of what is explored in these pages has less to do with sleep and more to do with Zen. This is not an intentional expansion of the subject matter, but simply a necessary part of the process: if the goal is to see sleep clearly on its own terms, then we must learn the art of seeing. That is what Zen tries to show us.

Of course, this approach can be used to address other problems and concerns, but for the purposes of this book, the application of Zen is mainly limited to the topic of sleep. Perhaps I will have whetted your appetite for more of this practice as it might relate to other problems or even to the Big Questions in life. There are numerous books available that treat Zen Buddhism more comprehensively, and with far more skill and insight that I have done here. Simply check your local bookstore or library.

How to Use This Book

It's important to not expect that anything "new" will be revealed in a Zen approach. At least not intellectually. Our Western self-help literature teaches us to "add skills," "internalize explanations," and "grasp key concepts." Such cognitive creations only take up space and requires mental effort. Because academic knowledge is ever increasing, we have been led to believe that understanding consists of adding knowledge rather than removing it. Or, if nothing is added, then we must at least replace or update it. Not here. Enlightenment transcends academics and "knowledge about."

The understanding depicted here is not just a matter of belief, as it is in other spiritual traditions and philosophies. To get the most out of this book, it will be necessary to give up thought and belief. Instead, take the time to search for the inmost meanings of the words used here. Set aside what you may automatically assume they mean. In a rather simplistic nutshell: Read the words. Search to find what the words refer to, whether they are pointing to your own assumptions or to a particular aspect of sleep. Once you find what the words refer to, which will take practice, maintain your observation without judgement. Therein lies the path to understanding.

It may seem at times that struggling to grasp the material in this book actually *increases* insomnia. Because these words challenge long established ways of thinking, it's likely to keep you up at night. But that doesn't mean it's not a journey worth taking. Sometimes you have to do what logically seems backwards, in order to move forward on a more substantial level.

You won't find an outline of step-by-step, easy-to-follow instructions to "a better night's sleep tonight" as you might in a more conventional self-help book. The process of discovery in this book takes us on a journey that spirals inward, with themes introduced and then recurring, their meaning becoming clearer as understanding grows. Some Zen teachers say that all they do is repeat the same thing to their students, over and over, in different ways. A similar process is involved here: all of these words refer to a single shift in understanding — a shift so subtle that it may require many different promptings before it is apprehended by our normal consciousness.

So the best approach to take is simply one that goes with the flow. Consider this a road trip, where you encounter the unexpected and you have the luxury of spending as much or as little time as you want at each attraction. Something particularly mysterious or enjoyable? Spend more time there. If you want to backtrack, feel free.

That said, you may feel an urge to flip ahead; however, the actual process of removing layers of misunderstanding about sleep is more easily accomplished if you first read this book cover to cover. In fact, it will be best not to proceed unless the issue at hand is well understood. In Zen, removing mental obstructions that cloud our vision is paramount. If we conduct our first, more basic observations as deeply and thoroughly as we can, the later, more difficult ones will be more penetrable.

Don't expect instant enlightenment, of course. Glimpsing reality through the fog of thinking takes time and practice. Often it requires repeatedly returning to earlier points that you assumed were understood. Thus, what might appear to be useless repetition of a particular theme in a more conventional book has, in fact, an important purpose in this one.

Along the way, you'll encounter terms referring to different aspects of what might be called a general sense of being conscious. While easily interchangeable, these words do carry subtle differences in meaning. "Consciousness" refers to the broadest sensation of oneself and one's surroundings, a kind of ongoing organic perception of our lives in our bodies and the larger environment. "Awareness," on the other hand, refers to our more specific sense of events in our environment — both outer and inner — and which often drifts about without our intention. For instance, I'm aware now of the touch of my hands on this book, a slight headache, now the feeling of my back on the chair, and now the sounds outside the window. "Attentiveness" is a more intentionally focused form of awareness, like the attention you are giving to these words. It too can be directed outward or inward. "Experience" is used quite broadly, to cover the overall impression that remains as the present becomes the past.

In this book, the term "mind" is used somewhat generically, referring to the part of our being that separates and categorizes all experiences. The "intellect" builds upon these divisions, creating a web of concepts and strategies. Finally, we'll refer most often to "the Thinker" (although usually not in very flattering terms), who generates a variety of mental distractions.

Holding on to all this terminology as you read is not as important as sensing the meaning from the context. In this way, *Zen and the Art of Sleep* is like a compass, pointing in the direction you need to travel. If, out of habit, you keep your gaze focused on the compass, reading as though the words themselves are important, then you'll have gone nowhere. After all, these words are just ink spots on paper. Take a moment now to fully grasp that fact. Don't "think" it. *See* it! What really matters is what you see and experience, beyond the reach of any book.

To facilitate this, you'll find a few exercises, called "Zen Practice" at the end of each chapter. Traditional Zen Practice, arising from a compassionate understanding of the intellect's ways, has as its goal a quiet and disciplined mind. While the goal here is somewhat different, the path to each is similar.

So grab a cup of coffee if you like (decaf, maybe?) and make yourself comfortable. Let's start with the obvious: why Zen?

Chapter 1

Why Zen?

Sleep has, for many of us, become mysterious and problematic. Despite our best efforts to control this part of our lives, nighttime can be a time of dread when we're unable to sleep. Insomniacs long to be free from the confusion and anxiety associated with what should be a pleasurable and rejuvenating experience. There may be a realization that one's own mind contributes to the unrest, but no easy solutions exist. Root causes are nowhere to be found.

The high rate of visits to doctors and sleep clinics, extensive use of medications, and frequent media coverage indicate that the problem of insomnia is getting worse in the general population. When the usual methods don't work particularly well, it makes sense to look for others, and that is the point at which many of us find ourselves in regard to sleep.

Religion offers little in the way of meaningful help. There may be general spiritual support in the form of prayer, which is used to address a wide range of human suffering. For the most part, sleepless nights are treated like any other troublesome part of life, and addressed within the conventions of a particular faith. Some schools of New Age thought occasionally speak to the issue of sleep, but only to theorize that dreams are actually journeys to other realms, or other unprofitable beliefs. There exists no specific religious ritual that has been proven to aid those in need of sleep.

Science has offered considerably more assistance to insomniacs, though not always with complete success. Mainstream medicine frames the phenomena of sleep as a biological function, and has to some degree succeeded in inducing or delaying sleep with medication and behavioral remedies. While the specialized field of sleep medicine has grown tremendously in recent years, no magic bullet has yet been developed.

Nonmedical treatments for insomnia, like those offered by mental health professionals, usually involve environmental and attitudinal adjustments. Clinical psychology leads the way in this arena, with exhortations to change your life and take control of problems. It would tell us that if we first clarify what our problems are — inner or outer, past, present, or anticipated ones — and then systematically resolve them, stresses and tensions will dissolve and our insomnia (and other troubles) will be fixed. Other schools of psychology teach clients to rethink conflicts, and to find new ways of thinking about things in general. But, as we know all too well, sleep can be particularly resistant to efforts to control it. And it couldn't care less what the experts have to say about it.

Likewise, sleep has a way of doing its own thing when the focus is turned toward the bedroom. Purchasing a new mattress, hiding the alarm clock, listening to soft music or sounds of nature, etc. are all attempts to bring forth that elusive rest. Sometimes these things work. There is certainly no harm in trying. Medication usually brings forth sleep quicker than other strategies, but not without its own potential problems. Unfortunately, no one strategy, alone or in unison with other changes, has shown itself to always aid those seeking rest.

Forcing change is a tradition in Western culture, and the fact that Zen requires no behavioral or cognitive change is problematic for a Western mind. "After all." the usual thinking goes, "if there is suffering then there must be a cause, and when we remove or modify that cause, the suffering will go away."

So in picking up this book for the first time, you most likely wondered, "What kind of solutions does Zen provide?" Your assumption might be that, since Zen is a particular philosophy, it must have a unique "spin" on sleep. In reality, Zen is about removing *all* manner of interpretation in order to replace concepts with direct experience. Sleep is just one of the many things we fail to understand because the mind has its own explanation — and that explanation is not the real thing. To answer the question "Why Zen?" is to clog the mind with yet another version of reality, to reinforce the Thinker's perspective: "It's only a matter of finding the 'right' way." But there is no right way: there is only how things *are*, which can rarely if ever be captured by a set of beliefs. How things really are is what a Zen approach hopes to reveal.

Your intellect, which we are calling The Thinker, will struggle with this. It wants Zen to have its own rationale, beliefs, and practices. Buddhism can provide rituals and intellectual byways that are able to accommodate the Thinker. However, in Buddhist traditions as in most others, these accommodations mostly act as distractions. There is no particular pathway to sleep espoused by Zen. So don't be afraid — allow your mind to protest.

We begin our journey not by surrendering to the Thinker, but by seeing beyond it. Asking "Why Zen?" appeals to the intellect. "Why Zen?" asks Zen to justify itself with arguments and rationales, and to appease academic types, this chapter will address the advantages of a Zen approach to the problem of insomnia. The more reflective query, however, is "Why the usual approaches?" That digs much deeper, confronting the Thinker's entrenched strategies, challenging it to prove that its ways are better. By examining where we already *are*, our hitherto unexamined beliefs about sleep will finally see the light of day.

Therein lies our freedom, because we will discover that intellect-based explanations of sleep have but a flimsy basis in reality. We will discover that anything not Zen, which is to say everything we *think* we know about sleep, is of questionable value. There may be much to occupy the mind, but none of it will cure our problem with sleep.

Alas, the Thinker will not loosen its grip until this becomes crystal clear. When our thought-based conceptions of sleep finally crumble under intense examination, we will be freed from false understandings. The true nature of slumber remains, to simply be experienced rather than explained. Therein lies our game plan.

Beyond the usual

Zen says that suffering is actually a result of the "usual thinking" we employ to explain and control our day-to-day experiences. In fact, *any* thinking, no matter how nontraditional, will only block the path to true understanding. Why? Put in the most fundamental terms, it's because there is far more to our existence than the reasoning process can grasp. We are a part of the universe, which is a vast and constantly evolving flow of energy, every moment giving birth to the next. The Thinker wants a beginning, a middle, an end, and a tidy summary. Yet our universe provides far too much unfolding information for the Thinker to process. A system of complex continuity can only be intuited with direct, moment-to-moment awareness of its continually changing contours. In this way, the potential exists for sleep to be experienced naturally, in the moment it arrives and as it unfolds — just as we experience every other moment throughout the day and throughout our lives — rather than analyzing it intellectually. Directly experiencing the flow gives us a more complete understanding than do the mind's stale recollections and groundless projections.

A clear vision of sleep is free from any attempts to encapsulate or analyze it. This is a type of understanding that exists on a different level than academic knowledge: it requires us to be in sync with the flow of life, without regard to the "how" or "why" of it. Right now this may seem too abstract, but that's because quiet reflection on the nature of things plays no role in contemporary Western culture. Yet this is exactly the approach needed for understanding sleep. The anguish of sleepless nights, barring the presence of an underlying medical condition, is for the most part a result of the Thinker's relentless need to analyze and control experience, rather than merely being present *with* it. Or so a Zen master would say.

The duty to sleep

One of the most common ways that the mind creates sleeplessness goes unnoticed: that is, the widespread tendency to place enormous significance on sleep. We do this without knowing why we do it, let alone what its consequences may be. Many, in fact, feel they have a "duty" to sleep. In reality, it is simply the dominant social standard to set aside time after sundown for rest. If it seems odd to be regarding sleep in an abstract social context, it's because we aren't used to examining the influence that social norms and assumptions have on our common day-to-day experiences. We aren't used to the self-examination required by Zen practice.

Social customs are simply ways of organizing group behavior. Conforming to social customs regarding sleep is an option but not an obligation. Sleeping, whether done alone or with others, is essentially a solitary experience: it is not required for anyone else's well being but our own. To attach a sense of duty to something that has no impact on others makes no sense. We may feel an obligation to sleep because of a vague apprehension that a lack of alertness during the day might have some kind of negative impact on our lives. If you look closely,

though, you'll see that it's not the amount of sleep we get that really affects us — it's our expectations of how others might react the next day that makes us anxious. We'll examine this particular misconception more thoroughly later in the book. For now, just recognize that social customs do not an obligation make. We humans have a propensity for missing the significance of truly important connections because we are anxiously looking in the wrong place. So warned the Buddha.

Discovering that there is no duty to sleep can bring comfort to those who have subconsciously believed otherwise. This is just a start, however: more insights are possible, provided we can identify and examine other spurious assumptions and test their validity against direct experience.

Sleep and success

If an employer wants an employee to be alert for their job, it isn't sleep per se that's at issue — it's job performance. Some people sleep very little and perform just fine at work. Albert Einstein, for example, never slept more than an hour or two at a time, but managed to do brilliant work all the same. On the other hand, some people sleep soundly all night and perform rather poorly at work. Clearly, it's our *performance* that matters, not the number of hours of sleep we get. Habit makes it difficult to give up our thought-based conjectures about what contributes to the successful outcome of human endeavors — even in the face of countless examples of sleepiness not impeding success, and even more examples of abject failure despite absolute alertness.

Perhaps the deeply held belief that a good night's rest is necessary for success the next day is simply incorrect. Could it be that rest is less important than other factors, such as skill and interest, along with situational specifics, that determine a particular outcome? After all, to err is human, as the saying goes. When sleep is given so much importance it becomes difficult to consider other factors. If anything that happens during the day has a relationship with the previous night's sleep, it's an assumed one.

The Thinker *believes* it is there because rest seems to bring alertness, and alertness seems to be a condition for success. Can we really infer causality here? Or are sleep, alertness, and success merely occurring in chronological order? Close observation reveals that sleep usually, but not always, precedes alertness, and alertness sometimes, but not always, precedes success.

More importantly, what exactly *is* success? If we strip away our usual mental associations and emotional reactions to the word itself, "success" (or the lack of it) is merely a human judgement about whether particular desired goals were met or not. The drama of planning, desires, and disappointments exists not in the real world, but in the mind. To someone struggling to climb the corporate ladder, the idea of success is as real as a mountaintop, yet, in fact, it's not real at all. Zen practice reveals this truth.

The Buddha said that observing the way things change will give us a more accurate view of reality than the static concepts of the intellect. Did he mean to imply that concepts are not reality? In other words, that human conventions like "necessity," "importance," and "success" aren't really *real?* Well, yes. Close observation reveals that they can't be seen, touched, or otherwise verified, and that the meanings we give them tend to vanish, reappear, and change over time. Constructs like these are born from the mind's desire to interpret and control everything around us, and do not physically exist — no more than little green men from Mars. Do we need any more proof that "necessity," "importance," and "success" aren't real? If something can't be verified in our daily life through direct experience, does it deserve to be called Real? With the status quo so embattled, the Thinker is protesting mightily. It's domain begins to be threatened when we first discover that our "Sleep is necessary for success" formula expresses little more than a customary belief.

Looking closely, we observe that our assumptions themselves change depending upon when we start and stop noticing the sequence of things. If daytime success always seems to come before restful nighttime slumber, would that mean that daytime success is necessary to sleep soundly? What is the difference between that interpretation, and the more common one that starts at night and ends at the end of the following work day? The two assumptions could be identical, except that they've been measured from arbitrarily selected points in time. Neither one is a particularly accurate view, since reality guarantees that things will always change from moment to moment.

To conclude: we can say that daytime success is not necessary for nighttime rest, because our direct experience has often shown us that rest comes even when daytime activities have not been particularly successful. And it's equally true to conclude that nighttime rest is not necessary for daytime success, because our experience has been that success has often come even when nighttime was not particularly restful. That is how it really happens, the Thinker and its beliefs notwithstanding.

Such mental aerobics are not intended for our entertainment, but rather to illuminate our problem. We may believe that sleep is necessary for success because of the way we look at it: that is, the way the mind looks at it. More devastating (to the Thinker) is that the way the mind sees things is often not even verifiable as real! By now the mind may be screaming in dissent, and loudness is its forte. But you don't have to give in. Better to get used to it. Later on, we'll explore how to manage a defrocked intellect.

Out of the box

For the next few days, observe the evolving quality of the following sequence, without thinking about or analyzing it: awake evolves to sleepy and to sleep, which shifts back to wakefulness. One quality becoming the next until it comes back full circle. This is what Buddha referred to when he said that observation of change gives us an accurate picture of reality. But what exactly is it that we're looking for in this sequence? We're beginning to observe the mutable nature of consciousness: the mind wants to intrude into this flow, labeling some sensations with the word "awake" and other sensations with the word "sleep." If we can refrain from this habitual labeling during our observation, we'll have our first significant clue that these states may not be separate events after all, but different manifestations of the same thing.

Our momentary glimpse of the changing nature of consciousness has already opened a new door, but it's still too early to enter. Seeing the whole instead of its parts is a profound shift in understanding. It takes time. Keep in mind just how out-of-the-box this new way of looking at what we call consciousness really is.

Freeing ourselves from the self-imposed conceptual boundaries like "necessity" and "importance" is crucial if we are to see the whole picture. Our mental frameworks, which perpetuate the illusion of parts, may seem to give us a measure of security. In the end, however, our ability to accurately perceive the subject at hand is clouded. Therefore, the challenge is not to "obtain" sleep per se, but to escape from how we perceive sleep.

Individuals vary widely when it comes to their ability to identify and set aside their cognitive beliefs. The more a particular idea has been reinforced by others, such as sleep's "importance," the harder it is to question it. We may have emotional investments in certain opinions, and some ideas may be connected to others in a kind of domino arrangement so that when one falls, the others topple, too. Our emotional need for stability may seem to preclude honest self-reflection. But the opportunity for insight still exists: we have many occasions and plenty of time to test our beliefs against direct experience. The personal journey into sleep-enlightenment is more a one-step-forward, two-steps-back process, way back to the long-forgotten state before sleep was a problem. Zen does not offer a ten-step program to achieve good sleep, or anything else for that matter. But when you master its logic, new directions and insights are possible.

The shape of Zen

A Zen approach requires no background or skill. There are no prerequisites for self-examination, a practice that Buddhists have done for centuries. But self-examination lies largely outside the Western cultural model, which defines knowledge as derived from the external world, not originating inside oneself. Religious salvation or liberation have usually been construed as being achieved through personal accomplishment or the intervention of a transcendent deity. Therefore, Westerners who are unfamiliar with Eastern philosophy may believe Buddhism in general and Zen in particular to be enigmatic or inaccessible. Some pundits have indeed complicated our understanding of Zen with references to the cryptic riddles of Zen masters, and multiple schools of interpretation. But, fundamentally, Zen is quite simple.

Zen is focused on discovering how your own mind creates unnecessary suffering. This is also a primary goal of clinical psychology, and in some respects they overlap. But Zen offers no analysis or method for seeing how one's mind operates: it teaches clear seeing and little else. The resulting departure of incorrect beliefs and the suffering that accompanies them is merely a consequence of this unhindered vision.

Some say that Zen's continual scrutiny of the mind can become a counterproductive obsession with suffering, yet we do need to uncover the everyday messes that we have devised for ourselves. From the point of view that trouble is best dealt with by denial or avoidance, the examination of suffering could appear unhealthy: if focusing elsewhere means misery is more easily endured, why not? For the simple reason that our miseries will still exist, and one way or another, they will continue to demand our attention in uncomfortable ways.

Another common misunderstanding of Zen is that it promotes an escape from everyday life because its focus is inward. In truth, it does quite the opposite: Zen requires an up-close examination of sometimes painful realties. Rather than being escapist, it is a here-and-now approach, challenging us to ask questions like, "What insights can I gain from directly experiencing this moment?" and "Where did I get this particular assumption?" and "What is the result of my holding this belief?" Zen asks for our willingness to look unflinchingly at how we distort our world, and to compare that with how the world actually is. It's a journey into understanding oneself, which may well be the most sane endeavor a person can ever undertake.

A Zen approach to insomnia is fundamentally rational. It is rational because Zen is not a religion: there is no deity or belief system involved. Zen requires no leap of faith. For societies anchored in Judeo-Christian traditions, the absence of doctrines can be unsettling, signaling a lack of credibility. We assume that anything of value to our individual growth must have some element of faith or belief. There is no answer to that, except to say that Zen is not a faith-based philosophy. It suggests, in fact, that we examine faith and belief themselves. No framework exists to promote any particular beliefs. Thus, you will find no theory of sleep within these pages. Although the mind is discussed, Zen does not take up residence there, as many religions do.

Contemporary Buddhists may adopt Asian modes of dress and behavior and spend time meditating and performing ceremonies in an attempt to gain inner wisdom. But this kind of cultural posturing is quite unnecessary.

A Zen approach to sleep is readily accessible. It requires no money or materials, and there are no scriptures to learn or skills to acquire. Ironically, this can make it especially difficult for a Western mind to credit, because we're taught to believe that wisdom is attained only through external efforts and issuing from some external source, replete with texts and ritual paraphernalia. If learning doesn't come from outside of us, then where *does* it come from? The Buddha said (and it bears repeating): "It comes from your own direct observation."

As a beginning step, simply verify for yourself that the "duty to sleep" and the importance you place on it are products of your mind's tendency to assume a dominant role; they are not actual things that you can directly verify. It may be the nature of the intellect to form concepts and theories, but is there any reason to place direct observation in a subordinate position? The Buddha said that a mind given free reign to jump on the conceptual bandwagon, without ever looking at reality itself, is a messy mind, and such a mind is bound to cause turmoil and suffering. Zen will challenge you to look at what you are doing and what the alternatives are, as we have already begun to do.

Understanding sleep is entirely possible if you are willing to open your eyes. You don't need to suspend disbelief, as though you are reading fiction or watching a movie. Indeed, the ways you may already be thinking about sleep may require a healthy dose of skepticism. Do they accurately reflect your own experiences? Zen doesn't ask you to accept anything at face value. It asks you to test the waters of reality and see for yourself.

Don't dismiss the challenges presented here without first testing their validity; responsibility for your own situation, after all, lies with you. It's all optional, of course, but the fact that you're reading this book indicates that you're on a quest. All of what you have read so far could very well be a bunch of hooey — and probably is, according to the Thinker. Yet beyond the veto of the rational mind lies something far more valuable: the real nature of things. Quietly observe the location of your awareness for a moment: what are you paying attention to right now? That may seem fairly easy, but it takes courage to stop thinking and start looking.

We are beginning to see that this approach to sleep has no formal structure, and because there is no "path" per se — other than your own individual path — there are no guideposts. And because there are no stages, but rather a burrowing through our layers of thought, there can be no common yardstick of progress. We either see our own thoughts as they relate to the larger picture, then assess their validity, or we don't. Concepts such as "progress" and "success" don't belong in this endeavor. Sleep is not a contest.

This is different from suppressing, replacing, or changing our beliefs. We must become comfortable with the kind of intellectual emptiness that can result from rejecting a long-held perspective. Hundreds of wise people over the ages have told us that to be mistaken is the human condition. We are better off when we humbly acknowledge that and learn to live with it. While our cognitive world may feel slighted, our spiritual and intuitive world will grow richer as our insight develops.

In the largest sense, the strongest basis for a meaningful understanding of the human condition is unwavering self-knowledge. Knowledge obtained this way offers the scholarly world a purpose and context within which truly worthwhile progress is possible. When it's not informed by an understanding of the true nature of our being, factual knowledge serves no real purpose and often leads to harmful undertakings.

It's because we all have a working knowledge of hunger that, over time, people have learned to develop and share the skills needed to grow food so that others don't go hungry. Likewise, we've developed the technical knowledge to explain sleep in physiological terms. But few of us possess insights derived from direct experience of sleep which could be used to help others in need. That's because we've been looking at the wrong kind of knowledge. Slumber lies outside our ability to explain or control: we need the freedom to experience it naturally, free from the Thinker's hectoring voice. Zen practice offers that opportunity.

The heart of Zen

At the heart of Zen is the observation that life will always escape our mind's attempts to quantify and qualify it. Reality just doesn't fit inside the mind. There's nothing inherently wrong about the way the intellect sees things, it's just that these constructs will always remain just what they are: ideas, not reality.

This doesn't mean that ideas serve no purpose. Concepts can be valuable and deserve respect — they are our best helpers with certain types of problem-solving. This concession might appear to contradict Zen's stated goal of freeing us from the Thinker's distortions. Not so. Just bear in mind that the intellect's version of something is not the *only* version, and certainly not the most complete one. It's when we fail to see the forest for the trees that problems arise. An expert will tell you which tree is an elm, a birch, or a fir. And an expert will tell you their ages, and how the surrounding ecosystem has affected their growth. But an expert cannot give you the experience of the beautiful woods. Only you can do that.

Appreciating the beauty and magnificence of an ancient redwood tree is the kind of "seeing" that Zen is after. There exists an essence, a completely nonrational understanding of such a grand work of nature. One stands in awe, touching the bark that extends upward to the sky. It is *directly experienced*, free from any attempts by the mind to capture its nature with thoughts. A small child gazing up at the redwood experiences the true nature of that tree far better than the most educated arborist whose mind is filled with facts and figures. The academic is blind while the child can see. The tree enlightens with a meaning and depth far beyond the academic knowledge of the most comprehensive textbook on trees.

This is easy to understand: a description of an ancient redwood tree is a poor substitute for directly experiencing the real thing. In fact it can prevent us from experiencing the real thing if we don't know such a possibility exists. But it bears repeating: this does not mean academic knowledge is worthless. The Buddha talked extensively about becoming mind-free, but he never said to stop thinking completely. He simply said to be wary of what you think, examine your mind, and do not let it control you. Spend most of your time taking delight in the things around you by directly experiencing the moment.

This way of lucid perception, referred to so often here and in other books on Zen, can only be hinted at. No language or method exists to capture it with words. "Seeing" reality is not exactly a matter of over-emphasizing your physical senses, although that can be one aspect of it. "Seeing" happens in that moment when a vital connection to everything in the whole situation is felt, making it utterly transparent and eminently workable. This book is an attempt to point the way to that dynamic perception in the realm of what we call sleep.

Zen Practice

Identify any assumptions you had about Zen. After reading this chapter, how have they changed?

Observe how you begin the process of self-examination. What feelings and/or thoughts come up?

Patiently watch your intellect protest as its ways are called into question.

Locate the "importance" that the mind puts on sleep. Now try to respect that, without necessarily giving it any power.

Chapter 2

Looking at Sleep

Having glimpsed the potential of what might lie beyond the reasoning mind, hopefully we are encouraged to keep looking. The Buddha's wisdom came from his realization that it was the mind that blinded him to reality, and the fact that the whole picture is not readily apparent to us now indicates that something is clouding our vision. Before a clearer picture of sleep's true nature can emerge, we must understand the intellect and other forces that have influenced us. This isn't an attempt to completely obliterate how our minds view sleep; rather, like the Buddha, we want to uncover our personal beliefs about sleep so as to not be blinded by them.

Cultural views of sleep

Our culture treats sleep as though it's a fairly straightforward phenomenon. Sleep is assigned a particular time, usually at night, and a particular place, normally the bedroom. One thing that the Culture of Sleep avoids is the key question of why we sleep at all, because there is no easy answer. Beyond polite references, like

"How did you sleep?," few people discuss the mysterious nature of slumber. Should we continue to pretend that we understand sleep? Perhaps, if one is sleepy, then sleep "makes sense." But when we cannot sleep, the question returns of why we sleep in the first place.

Such is the nature of the mind. It wants to know the how and why of everything. Experiencing an inability to "do" something always leads to a search for whatever is needed to "do" the thing in question. Taken further, the question arises of why we must "do" whatever it is, in the first place. Thus, when it comes to sleep, reasoning always returns to square one, the "why" of it.

The intellect can become demanding on this point, which presents a problem: we just don't have the kind of information that would satisfy the Thinker. As a species, we strive to understand our existence, and when something as ordinary as sleep fails to succumb to our investigations, perplexity ensues. It may be, however, that a less-than-perfect relationship with sleep is not only natural, but inevitable.

It's not socially acceptable to admit that our experience with sleep might be frightening, although not wanting to lose control is perfectly understandable. In fact, striving to remain conscious makes far more sense than willingly giving up control. In this way, the phenomenon we call insomnia is perhaps just a protective assertion against the loss of consciousness. Such a response could be seen as perfectly natural, rather than as a disorder of some kind. If you find yourself rebelling against the approach of sleepiness, why not appreciate that? Protecting the sovereignty of your awareness could be a good thing. For now, give yourself permission to rebel against sleep: the issues of control, choice, and responsibility will be explored more thoroughly later in this book.

Unfortunately, the academic term "insomnia" carries a negative value judgement. Our society bestows approval on the nightly act of going to bed and submission to sleep. Sleep is the goal, the Good, and the desire to remain awake and conscious at night earns a measure of disapproval. This is a carryover from a time when, as children, we were expected to be good little boys and girls who go right to sleep at the appropriate time. This expectation is no longer verbalized to adults, but the social and psychological vestiges remain.

Still, sleep arrives or not on its own schedule. Usually it comes in the evening, as expected. When sleep happens outside the culturally prescribed time, taking us by surprise, we are said to "nod off." Or, if we consciously permit ourselves to sleep during the day, we call it a "nap." Whatever labels we choose, it makes little sense to create a set of social values about something over which we have little control. The only things we *can* control when it comes to sleep are the meanings we assign to it and the way we respond upon its arrival. We might accommodate sleepy feelings when they come. Or we might not. Coloring sleep's arrival with the hues of morality serves only to muddle our understanding. There is no "should" or "shouldn't" — yet the expectation to surrender (or not) on cue still exists.

There are also hidden social meanings attributed to the state we call "sleepy." If it's the result of having been awake too long, we say that sleep is needed and the individual should go to bed. Or it might be that our sleepiness results from having already enjoyed the natural state of slumber for a long time, and wishing for it to continue as long as possible. Such idleness is often disapproved of, and we say that the individual has slept too much: they should wake up, get those chores done! Each admonition carries with it a message for the individual to somehow take responsibility for their state of consciousness.

This message to take control implies that there's a "right" amount of sleep to be had. It also implies that one can easily begin to sleep if necessary, or quickly wake up if one has had enough. And it suggests that being in some middle state between slumber and wakefulness is not a legitimate place to be. Most importantly, it reinforces the notion that sleep is an *action* that one has control over, and that infers *ability* is somehow involved. But the real decision involved is whether or not to accommodate sleep when it comes.

Yet sleep is not like other social imperatives. To even call sleep a "demand" is somewhat misleading, because sleep doesn't ask you to *do* anything. But it can be so adamant in its request for you to *stop* everything that it almost feels like a demand, and not all of us find it easy to oblige.

The invitation to sleep

Not everyone wants to accept sleep's invitation. After all, there may be better things to do than lose awareness of the external world and enter another realm. For some insomniacs, the whole process can be frightening: no longer surrounded by what is familiar, the onset of sleep means not knowing what is to come. Those who surrender are not necessarily smarter than those who don't. Perhaps, like newborns, they simply don't know any better.

For those who have trouble with sleep, the ideal world would be one where this uninvited visitor never knocks at the door. Imagine the extra time we'd have for ourselves, how much more could be accomplished if the boundaries between day and night were allowed to blur. And more importantly, there would no longer be a struggle at night.

Someone may say they "want" sleep, but that's because this visitor is *making them sleepy*. When we say that we "crave" sleep, what are we really saying? Perhaps only that we want to surrender to sleep instead of making the effort to resist it. Or maybe we want not to sleep but to escape consciousness. Often people who are depressed have a particularly good relationship with sleep because awareness is too painful — they happily abandon themselves. Others sometimes prefer to float halfway between slumber and waking, with no particular desire to be elsewhere.

If your soul could speak, it would probably say something like this: "For a certain number of hours each night, I raise the white flag and succumb to another power that, in essence, reaches inside me and turns the switch to Off. I relinquish myself entirely and enter nothingness, except for the dreams that remind me of my daytime world. I give up my present world of conscious awareness with the knowledge that in a short time I shall get it back again. That is my choice. That is my sweet surrender."

Meeting sleep's arrival like this, with a conscious decision, could be a good response for those of us who fear the loss of control that sleep suggests. As awareness diminishes, we could put aside our assumptions and fears and make a friendly connection. Just as it takes time for a new acquaintance to become a trusted friend, it can take time to become familiar and comfortable with this visitor who takes us to another place.

The feeling of sleep

When sleepiness first appears as a diminishing of our awareness of the external world, why not find the pleasure in those feelings? This pleasure is an effortless one, very much like floating where the tide takes you. It is a movement that carries you, with no force. You are merely along for the ride. Some people find actual physical movement to be sleep-inducing. Bus or train trips can be good venues for getting to know sleep.

For newborns, being rocked has a similar effect. Adults who want to understand sleep must become comfortable with being moved just like an infant. This doesn't necessarily imply being rocked to sleep by another person; it does mean allowing something else to move you from one place to another. The next time you are on a road trip with a friend, excuse yourself to the back seat for a short nap. Whether sleep actually comes or not doesn't matter. What does matter is the opportunity to relax while the change from here to there is done for you. Getting from point A to point B is not your responsibility. No demands intrude on your awareness, so you can safely drift away.

In fact, in sleep there are no demands at all. Sleep is like a return to the liquid womb where no duties exist. Complete freedom from responsibility. And no light, no sound, no activity. Sleep, unconsciousness, is the place you inhabited before anything else. When all that existed was the Great Beyond. A sense of that, beyond any rational explanation of it, can be cultivated from memory. Of all the places in the world, none is more secure, inviting, and safe than this place. Sleep seeks you out to protect you, just like a mother's womb. It envelopes you in security, cradling you in a cocoon far removed from the outside world. That, without interruption from the Thinker, is how it *feels*.

Remembering sleep

Some people can remember their very early childhood years, when sleep was simple and natural. Much of life at that stage is like that. Choices are limited, and "personal empowerment" unknown. Modern life for adults, on the other hand, requires considerable skill and responsibility. So it becomes necessary to go backwards in time to the very beginning. A good deal of early life is spent sleeping. Sleep is our starting point; only later does awareness of ourselves develop. Now is a good time to see if a memory of that original domain is buried somewhere inside. See if you can remember that sense of nothingness. Before there was anything to remember. The mind will protest, and may even fear going in that direction. But this sense of nothingness comes from an original sense of peace and security in the womb. Before anything else was even known.

On an intuitive level, letting go of the external world is an act of relinquishing control. People who surrender to sleep willingly do so because they know the pleasure it brings, and their response to sleep's invitation is effortless. For the rest of us, there's no hurry to get to that level of intuitive acceptance. We have many opportunities to sense the arrival of sleep and slowly explore surrender.

In a sense, adults have to start over, relearning how to accommodate something that doesn't make sense intellectually. Because adults tend to cater to the intellect, if something doesn't register mentally, it often doesn't register all. How can you recognize "nothingness ?" Newborns have nine months of practice at literally doing nothing; adults have untold years of forced capitulation to everything modern society throws at us. Perhaps if one could escape civilization and live worry-free on an island paradise, then one could become reacquainted with sleep.

Most of us have experienced periods in our lives when we found ourselves sleeping effortlessly. Usually this occurred when there were no demands on our time, and we somehow found our way to a place of deep peace. It might have happened on vacation, or perhaps a long weekend. Remembering what the luxury of that release felt like can be a sign of what to look for when searching for a grounding in sleep.

Unfortunately, few of us enjoy a continuous vacation; day-to-day existence is much more challenging. If many of the demands on us are adversarial in nature, then we tend to look upon changes in awareness (like falling asleep) in the same way. But unlike a client or colleague, slumber cannot be convinced to take less than what it's asking for. It wants it all — at least that is how the Thinker sees it. Sleep is something that will keep coming around for more until it claims all of your awareness. If you offer it something less than full submission, sleep will only continue to pester you.

Relating to Sleep

Drowsiness can be like a relentless mosquito that keeps buzzing around until it finally gets its fill of blood, then flies off. If you brush it away, it keeps coming back. If you let it take what it wants, it will leave you alone, but only for a while. Eventually it will come back for more of the same.

Those who enjoyably submit to sleep might shudder at such an unpleasant analogy. However, this is not written for those individuals, but for the rest of us who encounter sleep with even more dread than a nagging mosquito. Because no long-lasting sleep-repellent exists, sleep-avoiders must somehow come to terms with allowing this uninvited guest to feast upon awareness.

If you've ever had a mosquito land on your skin and begin its work, you are immediately confronted with choices — not only whether to allow the mosquito to proceed, but also choices about your mental and emotional reactions. If you believe a mosquito bite is deadly, then fear will overcome you. That's the Thinker (and its companion, emotional reactivity) doing its job.

It's the Thinker who perceives sleep as something separate from itself, like a raiding mosquito. Would the Buddha have worried about slumber stealing his consciousness? Quite the contrary: the Buddha saw that sleep is nothing but another form of consciousness, so there is nothing to be taken away. Can you point to or directly experience that which is "taken away" by sleep, and that which does the taking? The larger picture will gradually reveal itself, so be patient.

How each of us responds to sleep reflects our own particular relationship with it. We spend far more time examining our relationships with other people, yet sleep is a life-long relationship that surely deserves the same careful attention. At the beginning of life, we seem to have had the best possible relationship with this companion. What went wrong?

In fact, there is no "right" or "wrong" way to relate to sleep. After all, we have the perfect right to approach our relationships with others in uniquely different ways. From the Zen point of view, the ideal relationship is one that respects the true nature of each party; therefore, cultivating a positive relationship with sleep means permitting it to be whatever it is. And this isn't a question of skill. To sleep like a baby is indeed to have a very accommodating relationship with sleep, and babies are usually not considered more skillful than adults. Maybe we've simply become too busy as adults to maintain a trusting relationship with this part of life.

Too often, we approach the arrival of sleep the same way we approach a person whom we're unsure about, with caution and one eye on the door. This might be normal behavior with regard to an unknown visitor, but it is counterproductive when it comes to sleep. Trust has to be an inherent part of this relationship. There can be no search for power, no maneuvering to gain the upper hand that characterizes so many human relationships. Constantly strategizing in an attempt to control "the other" precludes any possibility of allowing oneself to be vulnerable — which plainly doesn't work with sleep.

Now let's briefly return to the question of why must we sleep in the first place. We return to this question not to indulge the intellect, for that is the source of our problem. Rather, let's identify that moment when the answer to the question of why we sleep appears with sudden clarity and completeness. That moment is when one is sleepy and the profoundly satisfying answer that appears at that moment is "because it makes sense." Notice how the correct answer reveals itself not when asked by the Thinker, but when casually observed as one moment flows into the next. At that point it really isn't an answer, because there is no question. It's just an observation that sleep makes sense. Not until the Thinker intrudes does a question of "why" appear on the stage. In the meantime, as one comfortably moves along in the flow, sleep makes complete sense. The only thing that makes no sense is asking why.

Zen Practice

Contemplate how culture has influenced your relationship with sleep. Identify how deeply "shoulds" and "should nots" are rooted in your mind.

Become aware of your personal reactions to sleep's arrival. Do choices exist?

Pay attention to the inordinate amount of thinking done throughout the day. See any ways to mitigate that?

Chapter 3

Impeding the Flow

At this early point you may be wondering what exactly is the flow? While the mind will want to conceptualize it, there is no actual "thing" per se. The flow just refers to that state of being when there is no attempt to define, understand, control, or change the moment. "Going with the flow," so to speak!

Alas, such a state of free flow living has become increasingly difficult. Zen practice, with its emphasis on careful observation of the mind, helps identify the many ways we impede the flow.

Sleep in modern life

How does one integrate sleep into a day-to-day existence that has, for most of us, become unsuitable for rest and relaxation? A real challenge, indeed. Modern life is full of demands, triggering that mechanism which keeps us awake and alert. If we only needed to be awake for primitive natural activities, there would be less of a problem. Now we find ourselves stuck in a kind of adaptational wakefulness, continuously responding to a level of demand for which humans are not suited for.

This is not to say that, given the opportunity, an individual would do nothing but sleep, only waking to fulfill a few needs. But such a lucky individual would certainly find it much easier to escape the many influences that trigger wakefulness. Students of Zen play close attention to what they actually do, moment to moment, during the course of a day. Inevitably, they find that much of a routine day is spent dealing with various matters, material things, and assorted responsibilities. While some of our affairs certainly seem pressing, and may be for financial reasons, much of it is just insignificant noise. Acknowledging this often helps to lighten the load, relieving the pressure we feel to stay focused on the many details of daily life.

Not all pressures are insignificant, of course. Care giving can be especially demanding, which limits the opportunity many women have to relax and recharge. Taking care of children, parents, spouses, and bosses keeps the focus on others. Over time the important task of taking care of oneself can easily become a foreign concept. When one's only value, as defined by others, is helping others, then not doing so, even at night, may trigger feelings of guilt and/or a mental accounting of who-needs-what. And for any woman who doesn't feel valued in her waking state, the nothingness that fading consciousness brings can magnify feelings of aloneness.

There is also the impact of our commercial culture to consider. In the West, creating desires and satisfying them has, for economic reasons, become the dominant activity and therefore the primary point of reference for how many of us think. Living inside this framework of manufacturing and then satisfying cravings, we unconsciously conclude that sleep is like every other need so eloquently detailed in advertising. Pills, special bedding, and other methods are touted as ways to buy sleep. If it works just a little, then more of the same is tried. The Buddha warned that when we feed our desires, they grow, creating an ever-expanding cycle that has no end. This continuous preoccupation with cravings and the ensuing struggle to fulfill them only hinders us in our quest for sleep's true nature. Sleep requires no craving or satisfaction of craving: there is only the invitation to relax and stop attending to the clutter that surrounds us.

Medical and sociological experts affirm that insomnia is on the rise precisely because of all the clutter, and no one doubts that modern life has become stressful and complicated. On the surface, this argument certainly sounds plausible. But the type of stress we experience is, in fact, far less threatening than in the past. We may have a larger quantity of details to keep track of, and while this makes life more complicated, it doesn't necessarily make it more stressful. The pre-modern world was rife with famines, wars, plagues, invasions, and general anarchy. Dire poverty was the lot of most of humanity. Yet nowhere is there mention of widespread insomnia. Given the relative ease of life today — compared with the struggle to survive that our predecessors endured — this seems contradictory. Shouldn't there be less trouble sleeping today, not more?

How can we explain this paradox? As the Buddha would say: Just Look. And if we look, we find that we've created and are inhabiting the Age of Information, completely blind to the consequences for our psyche. The Buddha discovered that our awareness tends to take on the qualities of whatever it is focused on — in other words, we become what we give our attention to. So, if forty hours per week are spent thinking instead of performing physical activities in the real world, guess what becomes the normal mode of our awareness? That's right, thinking. Analyzing. Conceptualizing. Add to this all the responsibilities of modern life, and we find that our consciousness has become distorted. Life is reduced to an overwhelming number of concepts, the modern currency of social and intellectual exchange. Sleep as been transformed into just another concept, one of many, ready to be processed, checked off the list and filed away in the morning, to be thought about again much later in the day (at the appropriate time, of course — nighttime). In short, reality has been hijacked by the Thinker. What a fine recipe for insomnia.

There must be a way that people of average means can cope, some way to turn off not the arrival of sleep but the realm of thoughts and ideas that demand so much attention and distort our experiences of life. Perhaps we can't turn it off completely, but at least we can turn down the volume.

With a clearer view of our predicament, some small steps toward a less "mind-centric" way of living begin to emerge. One obvious measure is to mitigate those factors that require us to be hyper-alert and thinking. A change of employment or simplification of lifestyle may help. In other words, we can compromise and find a middle ground where the things that seem to urgently demand our mental attention are scaled down in significance, through changes in either our circumstances or perspective.

It's important to realize, however, that these kinds of answers are more like band-aids than real solutions, simply because its impossible to return to an earlier time when cognitive stuff hadn't yet overtaken direct experience. Modern life requires a "mind-centric" way of living in order to get by. So we need to dig deeper to realize the hazards of too much conceptualizing.

Sleep as a concept

We lay our initial trap with the misunderstanding that sleep is somehow an entity in and of itself. That's easy to do. Simply point to someone sleeping (a picture of a person in bed with their eyes closed will suffice) and say out loud, "That is sleep." Carefully observe that there are only two things that can be verified through direct experience in this scenario. First of all, visual evidence shows us a person. That is all our eyes tell us; we don't really know if that person is merely resting their eyes. Second, observe your mind creating the idea of "sleep" from visual, cultural, and memory cues. Notice how that concept is drawn not from anything external or real, but from the mind's repertoire of associations and labels — and the label "sleep" is used to indicate a person lying down with their eyes closed. This particular word is laden with meanings that have accumulated over the years through collective assumptions and a medical culture, finally coming to signify that such a scene constitutes sleep, a separate and significantly different state of being.

However, sleep itself can't be pointed to because sleep exists, apart from one's own experience, as nothing but a concept. If it were more than just a concept, you could see an actual entity with your eyes and touch it with your finger. Instead, Thinker creates this powerful idea which acts like a magnet, pulling everything its direction rather towards the actual experience that lies beyond the reach of ideas and words.

Likewise the idea of "awake" exists solely in the mind. Try looking at "awake,' touching it with a finger, or in some other way verifying that what we call "awake" is substantially more than just an idea. Yes, there is a particular form of consciousness that is characterized by a heightened awareness of surroundings. From that moment we create a label called "awake." But nowhere is there a separate thing. See how the mind tricks us? Later on we will explore the tendency of the mind to divide everything up into opposites and apply labels accordingly. For now, simply verify how the Thinker has hijacked what we observe about ourselves with a design that obscures its true nature of one continuous flow that takes many forms.

This most fundamental observation — that "asleep," like "awake," does not exist except in our minds — challenges common sense. Wouldn't it be logical to draw the conclusion that this entire book is one big contradiction? Here's a book about sleep that claims there is no such thing! Well, from the Thinker's perspective, that might be true. If sleep doesn't really exist, why is so much written about it in these pages?

This apparent contradiction occurs because there are two kinds of perspectives on sleep. Only one can be written about — the concept of sleep — and that's the one that doesn't exist in the real world. It's immaterial, a mind-thing, and can't be directly verified; it's not reality. The other perspective — how sleep really is — arises directly from our individual experience, and can only be hinted at with words. It's the real thing, deeply felt and intensely personal. Alas, it's the first view that blocks our vision of the second, so our time is spent exploring the domain where sleep doesn't really reside.

But if we can get comfortable with the fact that reality isn't conceptual (which the Thinker demands), and that truth is often a matter of perspective, then many doors will open for us. It means that we are willing to acknowledge that anything of the intellect will, as the Buddha discovered, tend to lead us away from the real thing. We won't allow the Thinker to abort our journey just because paradoxes abound — we'll continue, and ultimately discover the path that is most useful.

When the going gets tough, it's time to return to the Buddha's central message, that real value lies in the direct experience of the present moment rather than what we think about with our intellect. The Thinker will insist that the shifts in awareness are separate entities. Its business is to separate experiences into opposites. If there is a thing called "awake," there must be an opposite thing called "sleep."

Yet close examination reveals we misinterpret the various labels we give our consciousness as actual things themselves, never feeling the underlying continuity of how it all ebbs and flows in the first place. So instead of simply experiencing each moment as it changes, we study every nuance to further divide and quantify the various labels we apply to the experience. Few of us observe our minds as intently as Zen practice requires, so this long excursion may seem like repetition — and that's precisely what's needed to really observe. You look again, and again, and again. And one thing discovered is that all the attention given to labels is like shining a light into an academic black hole. Don't expect anything genuinely useful back. It's only a label.

If an intellectual approach leads us nowhere, at least we have some indication of where not to go. Remember that our goal is the big picture, that clear vision that sees beyond the illusion of parts. Can we directly observe sleep and simply see it as a different form of wakefulness? No, not yet — the way is not yet completely cleared. Thinker is still in the driver's seat.

After all, the experience of sleep exists, the intellect exclaims. It was only last night that sleep happened, right? Well, yes — the experience happened. Does that mean there is a separate entity at work, a thing that is not you? Close inspection reveals that nothing separate is there, except for the mere idea of sleep. The old way of looking at "sleep" — as something that comes to visit in order to take away something else called awareness — has suddenly lost its grip. That concept may still exist in the mind, but it no longer has to override direct experience: one continuous movement of awareness towards and away from the surroundings.

To glimpse this is to understand reality. If a person were to tell Buddha that they've experienced sleep, he would probably ask, "What exactly was experienced? If you can describe it with words, then you don't fully grasp its true nature." You are looking in the wrong place, hoodwinked by the Thinker.

Need sleep?

The pressure to obtain sleep, both internal and external, can become so great that it takes on the urgency of a "need." And when one "needs" sleep, the search for it is on. Effort comes into play, along with a host of different responses. Observe how a reactive situation triggers the body to become aroused — and there you are, lying in bed wide awake. This whole process takes place internally, but as far as the body's arousal mechanism is concerned, the situation is like any other crisis. The Thinker has fabricated an emergency from the idea of sleep, something that exists only in the mind. Does sleep fall into the same need category as food and personal safety? If so, little wonder we lie awake at night trying to secure this element vital to our well being. Or have we just become hopelessly ensnared in our mind's tendency to create stories, and forgotten that the nature of consciousness is such that it will move in the direction of what we call sleep if we just leave it alone?

For students of Zen, the concept of "need" is a tricky one. It is a uniquely human idea. When animals sleep, it's not because of any concept of "need." It's just part of their nature. Why are we so different? One obvious difference is that we have minds that relentlessly separate our experiences into categories and attach labels like "need" — and when something with that particular label goes missing, we panic. So we go about trying to force things to be the way we think they should be, never realizing that it is our divisive intellect that creates the suffering in the first place.

The next time you feel this kind of internal struggle raging, instead of focusing on what the mind says you "need," focus on your experience of the present moment. If you are awake when you are "not supposed to be," so what? The mind will immediately answer that question with a long list of "dire consequences." But you don't have to believe in these warnings and respond as though you are a servant to the Thinker — or, worse yet, panic as though you are facing a life-or-death crisis. Simply be in the moment. Allow all that internal talk of "need" to continue if it must, in the background, while keeping the larger part of your attention on the experience of life unfolding in your body and all around you.

And if habit-of-mind is too entrenched, don't worry. The flow, like water, can only be impeded. It can never be blocked entirely. At some point the direction will turn to sleep no matter what Thinker does. In the end, all that is required is patience. Sleep always happens eventually.

Zen Practice

Recognize the ways that modern life makes your day-to-day existence more "mind-centric" than necessary. Any way to re-focus on something in the real world?

Can you permit the intellect it's labels of "awake" and "asleep" without giving them too much significance?

What reactions occur when your mind sounds the "need sleep" alarm? Identify other possible reactions.

Chapter 4

Freeing the Flow

It is human nature to attempt to control our lives. Most of our thoughts, words, and actions are geared toward bringing about a particular outcome. Zen does not exactly counsel us to give up control: the Buddha's outrageous claim is that we never had it in the first place, and that our suffering occurs precisely because of the efforts we make to manufacture it. When we realize this, our struggles for control naturally diminish. The challenge, then, is to see things as they really are. If our notion of control over sleep is an illusion, then perhaps it is not worth clinging to.

How can we once and for all determine if our hopes for control are misguided? Again, the answer lies in simple, focused observation. Does sleep start or stop on command? Can you, at this very moment, go to sleep? When slumber does come, is it because you have requested it — or have you merely made yourself ready for it? Close examination will reveal that control over sleep is more a matter of how we wish things to be rather than how they really are.

Our need for control is often the result of fear. Sleep does entail the loss of consciousness, but is there really any danger in that? We can look closely to see if in fact any hazards exist. Be in the moment, and observe the arrival of slumber closely. Because we can find no real threat, perhaps it is our thoughts that create fear. Does the Thinker label loss of consciousness a "danger"? Such labeling is, after all, what the mind does best — its job, so to speak. Zen respects the function of the mind, but without necessarily giving it the final say. Can you actually see and point to any lurking danger as awareness begins to fade? If there is no direct observation of a threat, then the mind is simply mistaken. Don't bother to disagree when the Thinker sounds this warning — simply direct your attention towards the truth of what is happening.

It would be easy for the Thinker to begin its strategizing here, jumping to the conclusion that, if the inability to sleep is really an act of avoidance, insomnia can be "cured" by deprogramming our fearfulness and compulsion to control, then reprogramming ourselves to submit willingly to sleep. Notice how the intellect rushes to capture a solution the minute that a new angle is discovered! This maneuver may or may not be useful. Self-protection is not a simple personality trait that can be turned on and off like a light switch.

Have you ever tried to tell yourself to not feel hungry when you're hungry? This kind of command tends to have the opposite effect, usually making you focus even more on your hunger pains. If sleep is to ever become a natural experience, it cannot be dealt with in the context of self-

control. Trying to will yourself to give up opposition to sleep is a mental gymnastic, and will inevitably create more internal struggle. If you've ever tried, you know it can't be done.

Meeting sleep

The Buddha said that we can eliminate the need for such mind-games through the process of careful self-awareness. Place your attention in the present moment. Observe how the mind creates a "me" and then an "it" (sleep), and bestows upon the latter an aura of danger, or perhaps of some mysterious power that must somehow be confronted. The Buddha would be quick to point out that this is the usual conceptual battleground: the more power given to Thinker, the more suffering.

If you've been following along this far, you may have already figured out the next step: to experiment with meeting sleep on its own terms. This lies outside the realms of the Thinker's mental grappling, or scientific theorizing, or emotional longing for solutions. It could bring us the kind of intuitive understanding that infants possess. They are free of the adult framework that stipulates that sleep must somehow itself be a separate state to be analyzed and practiced.

For thinking adults, this means throwing in the towel. Conceding the defeat of reason is not easy. To think of meeting sleep on its own turf, with no guidelines or theories, is somewhat daunting. But it can be done. It involves starting in the present, on square one, with an open mind and without regard for anything you think you know about sleep.

On "not doing" sleep

When someone asks, "How did you sleep?" what are they inferring? They hold an assumption so widely accepted as fact that it's rarely questioned. Consider the key word "did." This word is the past tense of "do," and therein lies the error — we either consciously or subconsciously believe sleep to be something we "do."

On the surface, it seems true enough. Isn't it obvious that sleep is something a person "does"? We talk about sleep as though it were an activity, and our use of language reflects that: for example, our use of words like "inability" to describe not sleeping when it is desired. But this whole supposition is fundamentally false. Sleep is in fact a complete cessation of "doing." Look closely at your experience of sleep, just as a Zen Buddhist would. Point to the "doing" in sleep. If you can't, then how do you know it is there?

When sleep is mistakenly seen as an activity, then we optimistically assume that it can be improved with some type of skill-building exercises, which, as we have seen, don't work. There is no way to change these social misconstructions, and trying to force the realization that sleep is not "doing" into a cognitive format only creates a vacuum. But it is possible to directly experience the truth that sleep is essentially an inner invitation to "*stop* doing."

In the Zen tradition, there is a saying that "The right view is simply that view which is not any one particular view." This means an outlook not colored by beliefs, concepts, opinions, or ideals; it is a vision free from the mind's obstructions. To observe sleep without using the mind is to see clearly that there is no "doing" there. That is the "right view" the Buddha spoke of.

Sensing the reality that there is no "doing" in sleep is gradual. "Doing sleep" is an idea in the realm of the mind, while "not doing" describes the effortlessness of drifting towards sleep. Our modern lives have become so attuned to reacting to demands and achieving goals that there is no place for a request to simply stop all activity. Our memories and future speculations are made up of action and reaction, demand and fulfillment, deadline and detour. How often do we receive a message to simply *stop* everything we're doing and just *be*?

The next time someone asks, "How did you sleep?" pause for a moment and translate this assumption-based question to a more accurate reality-based one: "How did sleep *happen* to you?" From that perspective you can offer a real response, even if the questioner remains stuck in the fundamental misunderstanding that sleep is something one "does."

Of course, others around you might not see that sleep involves no activity. How could they? In the Information Age, when so much of our activity consists of mind-work, the very notion of "doing" usually implies cognitive effort, especially regarding things we associate with the mind, like sleep. This observation carries us one step beyond our earlier conclusions about the concept of sleep. We saw how the modern world increases the amount of time we spend thinking, thus turning the experience of sleep into a concept. Now that we have discovered the "doing" aspect of our trap, we notice how the concept of "doing sleep" compels us even further inward, away from reality — because "inward" is where much of our modern doing takes place. If most of our doing is not taking place "out there" in the world of direct experience, but instead "in here" — in the mind — we are dangerously close to irretrievably losing sight of reality altogether.

Moreover, we have lost the habit of simply *looking* outwardly or inwardly. Given the relatively small number of demands on our attention from the physical world compared with the enormous increase in demand to think and "figure it out," this is hardly surprising. As a result of no longer having time to look, our misconceptions feed on one another without detection. Our cognitive material tends to form snarled webs of relationships that block the natural flow. So it's worth repeating the advice that Buddha gave us: Open your eyes. Pay attention.

Dreams

Instead of falling into the same "doing" trap with dreams — as in, "What did you dream last night?" — let's take a step back and look only at what can actually be observed in the world of dreams. On a physiological level, electrical impulses flit through the brain, combining and recombining at varying magnitudes and intervals. The resulting dreams create an alternate realm that often parallels the external world. Certain conflicts based in our waking world may get worked out here in ways that seem bizarre to the conscious mind. In fact, none of the rules of the external world apply: dreamscape is a place where absolutely anything can happen.

The vivid realism of many dreams is evidence that, from an experiential point of view, the external world and the dream world are interchangeable: both are subjectively experienced as real time, authentic events. We see, hear, act, and feel in a dream. People refer to "good" or "bad" dreams. We all like a good dream, and nobody likes a bad dream. A good dream can leave us in a good mood, and a bad dream can do the opposite. This confirms — if we didn't already know — that we are living, feeling beings who are affected by all of the events in our experiential reality.

Assuming that you're awake right now, you might protest that dreams don't carry the same validity as events in your "real" waking life. Yet in the midst of intense dreaming, there is normally no awareness that the experience is a dream. And most of us have experienced that disconcerting stage of awakening when we're not exactly sure where we are, or if what we just experienced actually happened.

If any experience — in dreams or elsewhere — is simply too peculiar to be "real," we're tempted to conclude that it didn't happen. If it was plausible but unlikely, we'll probably cautiously investigate. Occasionally we may even register a memory from a dream as something that's actually happened to us, and become confused when external facts don't reflect what we believe took place. The final determination of a particular event's "realness" is made not in the moment of the experience itself, but in the domain of probabilities; our minds swiftly and instinctively calculates the chances of a thing actually having occurred the way it seemed to. So apparently we need the Thinker after all, to decide what side of the fence an experience falls on.

And this is a most worthwhile function of the intellect — as long as it doesn't destroy the freshness of our experience once the calculations begin. To label an event "a dream" alters the experience, erasing its potential pleasure or significance in the service of our adult minds' need for the safety of a well-categorized world — a world we can immediately understand, so that we can quickly move on to the next challenge, the next obligation. Prior to learning this mental routine, we viewed the world through the eyes of a child; each experience was as valid and worthwhile as any other. Dreams were no exception.

Now, as grown-ups, we often sweep the memory of a dream under the rug, and sometimes we can't even remember our dreams. But on some level we know that dreams have happened, that our mind simply turned inward and created its own world. When our consciousness returns to the external world, only fragments remain of what we experienced while submerged in that mysterious other world. Many of us experience our waking life the same way: the individual moments and events that made up our day are, by evening, either completely lost to us, or else have become a blur of half-remembered bits of light and sound and meaning, to perhaps re-emerge later on, in our dream-world.

And dreaming is not exclusively limited to the times we're asleep. Many people have daydreams, some of which are so potent that they drown out the external world. We don't normally completely withdraw our attention from the outer world during the day, but when we do, we'll call it a nap if it is short and deep enough. If we're sitting upright, with our eyes open and our mind turned inward, then we say we are daydreaming.

Daydreaming is not identical to night dreaming. Someone who is daydreaming can quickly refocus their attention outwards, either of their own volition or because of some external trigger — unlike the more lengthy process of waking up from a deep slumber. Still, the differences between sleep and awake are less absolute than we would believe. We're usually — but not always — unaware of the outside world when asleep, and usually — but not always — aware of the outside world when awake.

Individuals who are quietly daydreaming seldom disturb those around them. But what if a person is actively engaged in their dream-world encounter, but is also awake and interacting with their physical environment, perhaps mixing elements of both worlds together? Those who can't distinguish between the external and internal worlds are labeled "psychotic," because they seem to be reacting to things that don't exist. According to the experts, those things they're reacting to differ little from ordinary dreams, both daydreams and night-dreams, in terms of their content. What may be lacking is that mechanism that summons the Thinker, who can then make those crucial calculations that distinguish between the practical "real" world and mind-stuff.

Even in psychotic states there is still some awareness of the external world, since the individual is usually able to move about in their environment and make a few appropriate connections with people and situations, even while hallucinations are ongoing.

The fact that hallucinations are a frequent consequence of sleep deprivation suggests there is some connection between the experiences of night dreaming, day dreaming, and hallucinating. And now the Thinker *really* demands an explanation! What could the missing links be? As we've discovered, the mysteries of consciousness lie outside Thinker's domain, so the solution to this riddle, or the realization that the question is a misguided one, must come from direct experience. Can we sense the connections?

First, we've seen that all three types of dreaming can feel alike subjectively. In fact, close examination will reveal the events in those realms actually can feel just the same as events taking place during periods of ordinary waking consciousness. Because of this, there are times when we have doubts about which category a particular memory or perception belongs in, asking ourselves, "Was it only a dream?" or, "Did I really just see what I thought I saw?" Only deep, completely dreamless slumber feels qualitatively different — that being a sort of "non-experience." Aside from that, the fact is that all experiencing ebbs and flows with a remarkable quality of sameness. The Thinker may be frightened by this observation; it erases all the neat divisions we so carefully construct to divide up the many ways experience happens.

Whatever differences there may be come not from the experiences themselves, but from how we view them. Or more precisely, how the Thinker (and other Thinkers around us) views them. The mind's system of identification tells us not what is happening inside — where it all feels pretty much the same —

but more about where our body and awareness are located when a given experience takes place. So if we are tucked into bed, it's late at night, and we are suddenly aware of our bedroom, having just experienced somewhere else, the Thinker immediately jumps in to reassure us that "it was just a dream." When a similar "somewhere else" is experienced outside the context of sleep it gets labeled a hallucination. Perhaps psychosis is only dreaming that doesn't confine itself to appropriate times. And maybe the so called "healthy" individuals are those who dream only when society says they should, mostly at night and with no concurrent awareness of the external — and occasionally during the day when awake, but without any noticeable and inappropriate interactions with dream-stuff.

Why undertake this disconcerting examination of dreaming? In order to sense the underlying ebb and flow of it all. The Thinker will still want to know the "real significance" of dreams. But we have seen that significance is created by the mind because of its craving for meaning, an explanation, something rational to be guided by. If we have the courage to question this yearning, we find that it's not really our whole *being* that yearns, but just the intellect, a small part of ourselves. Verify this for yourself by *seeing* that the issue arises from the Thinker's demands for answers, rather than a real curiosity about dreaming itself.

We may have an occasional nightmare, but for the most part dreaming provides enjoyment — satisfactions very comparable to those we get from day-to-day living. A particularly good or interesting dream can be preserved for later enjoyment just like any other pleasant memory. If the Thinker is unsatisfied with its inability to find stable ground here, so what? Dreaming, after all, need not be subjected to intellectual analysis any more than what occurs during the daytime. Do we always try to investigate and classify our waking experiences? Of course not. The depth and fulfillment of our waking life can never be captured by intellectual explanations precisely because it's *experience*, not something conceptual. The latter misses the point of the former: both our dreaming and waking lives demand to be experienced, not packaged by the intellect. Is the time we spend dreaming so very different qualitatively than our hours spent awake?

The mind says absolutely! Dividing and labeling is its stock-in-trade. We'll take a closer look at this in the next chapter. For now, simply experiment with this other way of seeing. See if you can observe not separate, carefully labeled entity-events, but one continuously changing stream of consciousness. The flow. Our new, nonacademic understanding of the nature of sleep unfolds slowly. Our path is not a straight one, but rather one that continuously circles back to bring forward insights discovered earlier in the process. This reflects the start-and-go quality of enlightenment, which can occur with either slight changes in perspective or sudden exclamations of, "Eureka, I see!"

There will be times when, in using words to communicate, we must employ the language of the mind. Now that we've explored some of the big picture, the word "sleep" can begin to point to a place on the changing spectrum of consciousness. It may still be a word and a concept, but now it contains some nuance that reflects reality more accurately. Because the word itself carries much of the old cognitive baggage, as we continue our exploration and the word "sleep" occurs, try alternating between the two kinds of understandings, the conceptual and the reality of how it all flows.

Thinker will insist that an understanding not of its kind can't coexist side by side with its own. But with practice, both kinds of understandings can exist side by side. A particular perspective will, by its nature, be exclusive. Yet other perspectives have validity too.

Sleep Medicine

Is a Zen approach to sleep problems compatible with modern medicine? Absolutely. It may not appear that way because of the mind's tendency to divide and label. Thinker says if our approach is Eastern than anything Western has no place in our endeavors. We will further explore this habit of mind in the next chapter. For now, just be aware of this false dichotomy.

Zen, after all, isn't any one particular path. It is simply awareness of all the paths available. If something works then it works. Whether it comes from an Eastern or Western tradition matters little. That said, sleep medicine has its roots in science where the most valuable ally is thought. Therefore the inclination is to think. Too much of that and the intellect quickly changes from servant to master. As any introductory psychology student will tell you, the study of mental disorders leads inevitably to anxious self diagnosis.

Our challenge then, is to benefit from sleep medicine without being held hostage to it. If you decide to seek medical help, let your doctor worry about the minutia of diagnosis and treatment. Whatever value resides in the academics of it all exists for the benefit of professionals. For you, the flow between awake and asleep is intrinsically personal and subjective, an experience far richer and more nuanced than the viewpoint medicine provides. For a patient who normally wants as much information and education as possible, such a hands-off approach can feel like the wrong thing to do. And for other situations that may be true. But when it comes to insomnia, better to let the experts do all the thinking.

It can take courage to let the experts see things through the scientific paradigm, while letting your consciousness take whatever form it does. Seep (and awake for that matter) won't appear on anyone's command. Still, the practical advice and emotional support from a doctor can be invaluable. And sleep may present itself more easily given particular circumstances. So try everything your doctor suggests to see what might best unlock the flow between awake and asleep.

He or she will likely recommend various approaches. Stimulus control and sleep hygiene forms the basis for most treatment. Progressive muscle relaxation and biofeedback can help you reconnect to that earlier time when unwinding was easier. Medication can also be useful. A multi-disciplined approach might work best. For the most comprehensive and skilled help, visit a doctor certified by the American Board of Sleep Medicine.

And remember the famous Zen saying: "if you meet Buddha on the road, kill him." That isn't meant literally of course. It just means be cautious of anyone who claims to know more than you.

As awareness shifts

When awareness begins its cyclic shift away from the outer world, we call that experience "drowsy." This fatigue of mind causes less strife for our intellect than sleep does, probably because there still remains at least some awareness of the outer environment. But, we ask, why does awareness change direction in the first place? That is the Thinker, once again asking questions. All that we can observe, and thus all that matters — because reality is all that matters — is that this seems to be the fundamental nature of experience. It ebbs and flows.

Redefining what we call "getting drowsy" as "consciousness inevitably changing its direction, away from the external world" throws the Thinker for a loop. Indeed, even calling awareness a "stream that ebbs and flows" presents a problem. As we know, the mind wants everything to be static, fixed at a particular point in time at a particular place, and preferably amendable to being measured and categorized.

Because of their unceasing flux, most aspects of consciousness elude every attempt to explain them. Obviously, awareness exists — "it" is looking at this page at this very moment. This fact will register with the Thinker momentarily, but not for long. When awareness shifts, it is best described as a change in direction — not that this captures the process, for we know that reality cannot be captured with words. But the ongoing change in direction throughout the day, which inevitably brings us to the moment in time that we call "getting drowsy," is not in itself a problem — unless the Thinker makes it one.

How will it happen to me?

Deep within yourself, you've discovered that drowsiness and sleep are both events that happen whether you want them to or not. Again, observe the experience of drowsiness, this time on two levels. First, watch how awareness of the surroundings diminishes. This is a flow that, as we have discovered, is best left to its own devices. This shift in awareness requires no effort and poses no difficulty. Here is reality, the natural flow that Zen hopes to uncover.

Then go ahead and translate this same process into mind-speak: you notice that drowsiness comes to you, rather than being something you actively solicit. Try to find it, and it will hide. Try to avoid it, and it will eventually appear of its own accord. This is how the mind views the events in our lives, as separate entities interacting with one another, and often at odds. This is a reflection of our troubled relationship with whatever we consider to be both highly desirable and maddeningly elusive.

Our tendency to go with the mind-based version of sleep unfortunately obscures our deeper understanding of the former approach — which is not a "version" at all. Reality lies in the *experience*, beyond the reach of words. Slowly but surely, we can change the meaning of the words we use so they more accurately reflect reality, even if words are a poor substitute.

With these insights, you can begin to perceive sleep's true nature — or, more accurately, the true nature of consciousness in the form we label as sleep. A shift in the flow is not a separate and discrete "thing," despite what our minds might tell us. You may not see the whole picture yet, so this perspective could still seem perplexing. Keep at it. Reality will slowly reveal herself.

Try approaching bedtime tonight with the question, "How will sleep happen to me tonight?" Or for those who can already *see*, "How will consciousness shift direction tonight?" Perhaps drowsiness and then sleep will happen to you in a light, fleeting way, taking you through continual shifts and changes in your experience. Perhaps sleep will not visit you at all. Or maybe it will arrive with such speed that within a few minutes you are deep in slumber without being aware of the transition. To participate in sleep in this new way, all that you need to remember is this: However it happens is alright. How sleep arrives, as we have observed, is beyond your control. Tomorrow will arrive no matter what sleep chooses to do tonight. In the morning, plan to ask yourself, "How did sleep happen to me last night?" Understand that sleep *happens*, coming to visit you with or without an invitation. There is nothing for you to "do." You need not put out any welcome mat unless you want to.

A famous disciple of the Buddha said it best: To carry yourself forward and experience myriad things is delusion; That myriad things come forth and experience themselves is awakening. In other words, actively trying to capture an experience — or even looking for an explanation — only disrupts the natural flow of this moment to the next moment. There is nothing to "do" or "know" about sleep.

If, on the other hand, you view sleep in the usual way, as something separate from yourself that you're individually responsible for, as something you "do," then you won't be able

to accommodate an ever changing consciousness. Your mind's habitual patterns will ensure the focus remains on you, your reactions, your thoughts — particularly your concepts of sleep — instead of where it should be, on the present moment, which may or may not unfold the way you would like.

This new approach — to not take any particular approach — brings us into what is, at its heart, a relatively impersonal realm where there is no sense of a "you" as hunter and "sleep" as prey. But now that we have sensed the true nature of awareness — that it ebbs and flows on its own — we may know better.

We've covered quite a bit of ground in the last several chapters. By now you have a better sense of what a Zen approach to sleep is all about. If you look closely, you'll see that you have come further toward where you already are. Nothing has really changed, except your understanding. The rest of the journey isn't particularly arduous; it does, however, take persistence to realize the whole picture. In the next chapter, we'll be going where the Zen masters go. Feel free to take a break, before tackling the most impenetrable of truths.

Zen Practice

How rooted is the "responsibility for sleep" supposition?

Watch how the mind frames sleep as an activity or skill. Now compare that with how it really works.

Remember a favorite dream and how real it seemed. Now recall a similar event from your waking hours. Sense how similar both are.

When experiencing the ebb and flow, how does it feel? And how does it feel when the mind tries to separate, label and control?

Pay attention to your present level of alertness. Does it seem to be increasing, decreasing, or staying about the same? Formulate a response that doesn't contain a judgement ("that is bad"), comparing ("this is better than before"), or refers to you; for example, rather than "I'm tired," say "There is drowsiness now."

Chapter 5

Beyond a Self that Sleeps

To take oneself out of the picture and allow the flow of consciousness to unfold — without the motive to acquire sleep — might seem rather puzzling. The very purpose of reading this book is, after all, to obtain a good night's rest. How could we undertake this journey in order to heal our problems with sleep, only to end with the conclusion that we never needed to do so in the first place?

Because now we see our situation. Finally we understand the heart of the problem that the Buddha pointed out: it's not the various shifts in what we call waking and sleep that plague us, but our own intellect, the one small part of our being that we've permitted to overshadow our direct participation in reality. The path that leads us out of this situation takes time and practice. Zen offers a way to this freedom from the mind. Our objective, as we've said before, is not to eliminate or control the intellect, but rather to not be subjugated to it.

Dualizing

Mind-activity is like a one-way street — and it always leads to opposites. Try this thought-experiment. Think about temperature, and you'll end up thinking in terms of either hot or cold. Think about size, and you wind up with big or small. Think about consciousness, and you end up dividing it into either "awake" or "asleep."

A close examination of these concepts reveals that, in keeping with the mind's polarizing tendency, they will appear on the cognitive stage only in pairs. If you take away the idea of hot, there can be no cold. Take away big, and small disappears. And in the context of our particular discussion, we invariably define sleep by what it is not, namely "awake." By definition, a concept will always have an opposite, and the mind will always bounce between the two, unaware of the fluid nature of reality that lies outside. This small bit of insight can take us a long way towards freedom from the Thinker's habits.

There are, of course, different gradations between the two opposite poles of any given spectrum, but even those gray areas still exist entirely in the mind and so are susceptible to becoming polarized. Think for a moment about the "right size" of some article of clothing. That "rightness" of size is determined precisely by what it is not, namely too big or too small. We can permit the Thinker to do its assigned jobs — like making these kinds of comparisons — but we don't have to give up the deeper and more significant reality of the moment. Feel that sensation you call temperature, wear that article of clothing, and allow consciousness to go where it goes. These kinds of organic, nonintellectual connections to the larger world transcend anything the experts can offer. Their vision is that of the Thinker — everything reduced to parts that can be fiddled with in an attempt to improve performance.

The Illusion of Self

Because our deeper understandings doesn't consist of parts, there's nothing to fiddle with. Ultimate enlightenment in Zen — what every serious student attempts to realize — is the liberation from the illusion of self. This is an especially perplexing aim for Westerners because, as we have discovered, so much of modern activity involves a notion of "self" as either the instigator of action or the recipient of it. On various levels, especially socially, that mind-thing which we call "identity" carries tremendous weight. And on a day-to-day basis there is obviously someone who goes to work, cleans the bathroom, and tries to fall asleep at night. Right?

In the mind-realm, that's true. But if we take a step back in order to look at the larger picture, without assigning meanings to any one element, we can observe individual beings — emanating from the larger — going about in what they imagine to be their own private worlds, unaware that every so called "part" has "boundaries" only because awareness is so limited. The *all* — one continuous stream of which everything is connected to and affected by — can still be sensed, even though it cannot be registered intellectually.

Given the dualizing nature of the thinking mind, humans inevitably see the world in terms of in here versus out there. In this way, reality is seen through a warped lens that causes a feeling of profound separateness from the world. It's little surprise that people struggle with existential questions because of this illusion, often turning to religion for help. The fact that everything is interdependently connected, woven from the same fabric — no "in here" or "out there" — can be sensed only in the moment-to-moment flow of life. Each moment gives birth to the next. Our spiritual nature ensures we can sense our connection to the whole, even if words fail miserably to describe it. There is — in reality — no separate "self" to be either awake or asleep.

Prior to this realization, there is a separate, individual human body the mind claims is "mine." But can you identify any entity to which the body belongs? Where is the me in "mine"? Try simply pointing to yourself. Carefully observe that what has been pointed to is a human body, one small element of the all. Now try to point to "whose" body it is. *See?* It may take practice, but at the moment it becomes clear everything changes.

Look at a photograph of yourself at a very young age. Is that you? Hold that picture up in front of a mirror to compare it with your reflection. Although the mind will insist that it's you, observe the substantial differences. If the "you" in the picture is not the same "you" in the mirror, exactly where is that permanent "self" you insist upon? Bodies, being intrinsically a part of the all, continuously change like everything else. Change, after all, is the only constant. The Thinker takes the easy way out, and calls it "growing old."

Consider your name: it's a series of words, an idea that has been reinforced by a lifetime of social interactions. Say your name out loud. What has been voiced is, in reality, just a sound. Take a moment to grasp that fact. Don't "think it." *See* it! Yes, the meaning given this particular sound carries great significance. And the experience of being a separate individual is valuable, inevitable, and worthy of respect. But the serious student of Zen realizes it is an illusion.

New students of Zen are sometimes terrified at being unable to directly locate a "self" — until they realize what a blessing that is. Existential questions about birth, death, and the meaning of life all disappear when the truth is discerned amidst the illusion of self. One glimpse, and in an instant all the heavy questions about "my" purpose on this earth seem to vanish. As reality of no-self becomes more a day-to-day experience, remnants of these initial fears fade away. Here lies the intellect's ultimate trick. "I" was never there to begin with. That is why the Buddha is so often depicted giggling!

Yes, a body was born, or more accurately, that current which is the "all" sent forth another new stream, the separate identity of which is created by the mind. It might seem strange to look upon our human bodies simply as parts of the larger universe, because we've added so many meanings along the way in order to create a "self." And again, this is a necessary, valuable part of being social creatures. Our individual selves do exist, socially — just not within the larger reality that Zen shows us. Zen masters sleep — or don't sleep — peacefully because they're not saddled with concepts like "self" or "sleep."

The wisdom of children

In this way, Zen masters are like young children who have not yet developed a sense of self. Without this added burden, the flow of awareness from moment to moment proceeds unimpeded. At an early age, experiences are not seen as "separate" from the one who experiences them, precisely because there is no "self" to do the experiencing. That artificial division between the self and everything else is created later on in cognitive development. Adult minds will have trouble with this until the illusion of self is broken through. Then, what children already know can begin to take root.

It can be illuminating at this point to observe how the intellect might demand a full accounting of what exactly it is that children "already know," expecting it to be in a form that makes sense intellectually. Yet we have discovered that children's wisdom is inherently nonintellectual. It turns out that humans don't need any version of sleep, or a "self" for that matter, in order to get by.

The delightful flow of unobstructed consciousness manifests itself most easily in children. And why wouldn't it? New life, no matter the species, embodies energy and excitement. The satisfaction of being one with the world — not the social concept of the world that adults have, but the literal reality that children experience — makes the world an easy and even awesome place to live. An infinite number of influences gather together at one point in time and cause a young child to squeal with the sheer joy of it all. Later, this bundle of energy will change direction and quiet down. Constant change characterizes everything. Therein lies the flow.

For newborns, who sail right along in the flow, not the slightest bit of structure exists in consciousness. Once needs are met, it takes only seconds to fall asleep. Obviously there are no skills or understandings involved. If that were the case, older people would find sleep more easily than the very young.

For grown-ups, it takes considerable spiritual gumption to reconnect to that earlier era of enlightenment and in effect say to an over-indulged intellect, "Yes, keep on insisting there is a 'me' that 'does' sleep or waking" — and then proceed to connect with the flow of the moment, knowing that awareness will change direction on its own.

Letting go

Because the flow of awareness is in constant flux — the antithesis of the static world of the mind — it threatens the Thinker. This is a frequent challenge for those new at meditation. Quietly observing your awareness can be like watching a four-year-old: neither patient nor focused, awareness will always divert itself to something else, and from there to something else again. At some point, it will turn its focus away from the outside world altogether, which is another aspect of its elusive nature. While a Buddhist merely observes all the different aspects of this flow, the intellect wants none of it. And that is OK. The mind deserves the same compassion as a child deserves. Each operates in the only realm it can, doing the only thing it knows.

Still, for the Thinker, sleep is the last straw, completely eluding all attempts to define and control it. There will simply never be peace as far as the intellect is concerned. But, now that we're aware of the underlying reality of what we're observing, the frustrations of Thinker need not take on so much importance. Its ramblings need not interrupt the flow.

They might at first, of course. Relegating a part of ourselves that has always been in the driver's seat to the back seat requires some adjustment. The tendency will be for the Thinker to call the shots, so expect that thoughts about the awake-to-asleep spectrum will make an appearance in the evening and possibly in the morning, along with stern warnings about the "need" to move from one end of the spectrum to the other. Eventually, all this will become mere background noise, like a malfunctioning alarm system that, being impossible to fix, warrants no more attention. Over time, it can just be forgotten about.

As it turns out, securing sleep is a conceptual red herring. It's worth repeating; the Buddha warned long ago that the mind will create this kind of unnecessary suffering. Only by accurately perceiving our condition in the moment is enlightenment possible. Then we can make those first steps, however awkwardly, to assign the Thinker a more appropriate support role. This realignment of the chain of command becomes easier as one realizes the mind's limitations. Perhaps for making comparisons in the physical world, the mind's ability to capture a moment and then scrutinize and evaluate it is invaluable. For anything else — and there is considerably more — we need our deepest senses to tap into more substantial truths.

When the hard work of really seeing is finally accomplished, the mind quiets down and life begins to ebbs and flow freely, like it did in earlier times. Wakefulness and sleepiness really are part of the same moving stream. Within that flow will come an inevitable nighttime moment of drowsiness, a moment not so different from any other, free to proceed naturally and without effort.

Zen Practice

Observe the dual nature of thinking without judgement. Now sense reality unfolding well beyond such duality.

When "self" is finally seen as an illusion, what feelings come up? Can the fear be managed enough to continue looking?

Remember life at its beginnings, before the ideas of "you" and "sleep" arrived on stage. Cultivate that memory.

Conclusion

Enlightenment rarely happens on its own. It requires our consistent attention to the ways that the mind supersedes our deeper sense of being. Not that we want to reject the mind which, as we have discovered, has its own valuable roles. But we want to discern where a deeper understanding might be found. Given our tendency to accept mind-based concepts as the gospel truth, observing our world with "bare attention" — without any accompanying interpretations — may feel awkward. Rarely do we reflect on the simple but profound fact that "how things are is how things are," and that this elusive reality is our true starting point.

Remember that the "right view" of Zen is perspective-free. It inquires into everything, with no preconceptions or understandings of any kind. Because this approach of not taking any particular approach can initially seem so paradoxical, we started our journey with some introductory discussion of Zen Buddhism. And at first we were unable to locate a Zen explanation of sleep. Only gradually did we realize there was a deeper truth awaiting our discovery, one that didn't involve theories or interpretations.

We reached this insight by contrasting our mental baggage — such as our nagging sense of a "duty" to sleep — with a quiet observation of reality. Not only were there no obligations to be found, but all our assumed connections between sleep and success in daily life turned out to be spurious. This plunge into the deep end of Zen may have felt rather unsettling at the time, but it did show us the value and power of our own direct observations.

Having gotten our toes wet, we went on to examine how cultural influences have shaped our beliefs about sleep. Value judgments grow like weeds when it comes to this subject, and it was relatively easy to confirm how useless they are. Sleep, it turns out, comes on its own timetable and in its own way. What few choices we have about sleep seem to have more to do with how we accommodate the arrival of sleep than anything else.

Remembering how we accepted sleep when we were children, in an earlier time of trust, opened a valuable door. Then reflecting upon our present-time, adult relationship with sleep revealed opportunities for change. The overwhelming dominance of thinking and conceptualizing in our daily lives became clear. Slowly, we began to see our predicament.

Up to this point, we'd had only a few glimpses of the nature of the ebb and flow of consciousness. Having already begun to sense it, we knew in a new, nonacademic way that what we labeled "sleep" was simply a change in the flow. All moments have a remarkable underlying similarity.

Finally, the "right view" of Zen started to make sense. Having begun our journey with no particular approach, discarding our preconceptions along the way, it became possible to discover that what we were seeking moves along under its own power, requiring absolutely no participation by us. We now had a much clearer sense of the flow as something completely outside of our control, and manifested most comfortably when we stop "doing" sleep — or anything else.

Watching the various ways that the flow manifests itself led us to further insights. Artificial divisions between dreaming experience and normal day-to-day experience break down when we sense how similar they are. Consciousness may be constantly changing, but it all originates from the same stream, even if it flows differently at different times. This subtle perception, long in coming and completely contrary to the intellect, reflects how all divisions are illusions of the mind. Such immensely satisfying insights are the rewards for Zen practice.

Lastly, we touched on the most valuable potential of Zen, that of becoming selfless. While Zen Masters perceive this easily, others can still catch momentary glimpses — provided there is sufficient bravery to do so.

When observing that the source of our problem lies with the adult cognitive boundaries that separate the different manifestations of the flow, the Thinker is tempted to see it all as a new system to either believe or disbelieve. The Thinker will even want to create new concepts based on these observations, a sort of "Zen version" of sleep. In fact, it will be all but impossible to read this book and not have the mind formulate a "Zen Sleep Strategy." But, as has been discovered, a world view that is captured by a set of beliefs or concepts can never match reality itself, simply because reality is not frozen. Reasoning insists that essential truths can be captured within a particular framework, but that ignores our deeper intuitions, which sense the fluid and flexible nature of existence. The Buddha understood this, and saw how enlightenment flows only from direct, mind-free, moment-to-moment experience.

Therefore, we should be cautious about assuming that *Zen and the Art of Sleep* represents reality. This rather formless little tome, the pages of which offer neither academic explanations of sleep nor methodologies to "acquire" sleep, will act at best like a compass pointing in the right direction. No book can capture reality, because any explanation will, by the very fact that it is a construction of the mind, lack the validity of the real thing. Instead, *Zen and the Art of Sleep* offers a life raft across the rough waters of the intellect. Once on the other side, it is best to leave the raft behind. Otherwise the raft, simply a means to an end, may be confused with what matters — how things really are.

And at some point focusing on the experience called sleep will no longer be useful. Given its freedom, awareness flows along though its many forms rather freely, needing no particular attention, and certainly not constant monitoring. For once reality is seen, nothing much remains to be done, except perhaps just letting it all go.

Eventually this little book will have to be discarded. And that's when the art of sleep will be mastered. It's all very simple, really. Just go with the flow.

Printed in the United States
128051LV00004B/31/P